KETO DIET FOR BUSY PEOPLE

Guide To Cooking Easy ketogenic Recipes for Weight Loss and Stay Healthy

Snowie Danelle

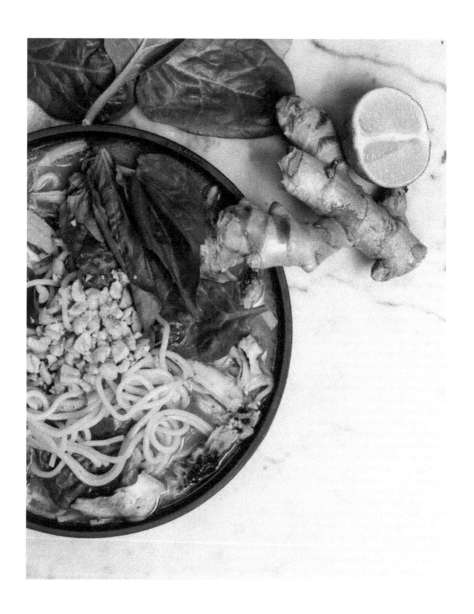

CONTENTS

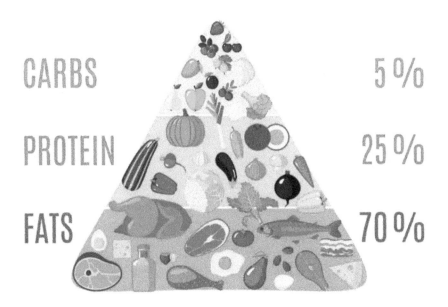

1. CAULIFLOWER CHEESECAKE

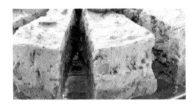

Preparation Time: 20 minutes

Cooking Time: 30 minutes

Servings: 6

Ingredients:

- 1 head of cauliflower (cut into florets)

- 2/3 cup of sour cream

- 4 oz. of cream cheese (softened)

- 1½ cup of cheddar cheese (shredded)

- 6 pieces of bacon (cooked and chopped)

- 1 tsp. of salt

- ½ tsp. of black pepper

- ¼ cup of green onion (chopped)

- ¼ tsp. of garlic powder

Kitchen Equipment:

- oven

- baking tray

- bowl

Directions:

1. Preheat the oven to 350°F.

2. Boil the cauliflower florets for 5 minutes.

3. In a separate bowl combine the cream cheese and sour cream. Mix well and add the cheddar cheese, bacon pieces, green onion, salt, pepper, and garlic powder.

4. Put the cauliflower florets into the bowl and combine with the sauce.

5. Put the cauliflower mix on the baking tray and bake for 15–20 minutes.

Nutrition: Carbohydrates 8g - **Protein** 15g - **Calories** 320

2. FISH CAKES

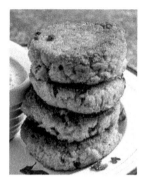

Preparation Time: 10 minutes

Cooking Time: 8 minutes

Servings: 6

Ingredients:

For Fish Cakes:

- 1 lb. of whitefish fillet (wild-caught)

- ¼ cup of cilantro leaves and stem

- ¼ tsp. of salt

- 1/8 tsp. of red chili flakes

- 2 garlic cloves (peeled)

- 2 tbsp. of avocado oil

Dipping Sauce:

- 2 avocados (peeled, pitted)

- 1 lemon (juiced)

- 1/8 tsp. of salt

- 2 tbsp. of water

Kitchen Equipment:

- food processor

- large skillet pan

- blender

Directions:

1. Prepare the fish cakes and for this, place all the ingredients for the cake in a food processor, except for oil, and pulse for 1 to 2 minutes until evenly combined.

2. Then take a large skillet pan, place it on medium-high heat, add oil and leave until hot.

3. Shape the fish cake mixture into six patties, then add them into the heated pan in a single layer and cook for 4 minutes per side or until

thoroughly cooked and golden brown.

4. When done, transfer fish patties to a plate lined with paper towels and let them rest until cooled.

5. Meanwhile, prepare the sauce and for this, place all the ingredients for the dip in a blender and pulse for 1 minute until smooth and creamy.

6. Place cooled fish cakes in batches in the meal prep glass containers and stock in the refrigerator for up to 5 days.

7. When ready to serve, microwave the fish cakes in their glass container for 1 to 2 minutes or until hot.

Nutrition:

Calories: 69

Fat: 6.5g

Protein: 1.1g

3. PORTOBELLO MUSHROOM PIZZA

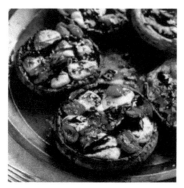

Gluten Free, Nut Free

Preparation Time: 15 minutes

Cooking Time: 5 minutes

Servings: 4

Ingredients:

- 4 large portobello mushrooms (stems removed)

- ¼ cup of olive oil

- 1 teaspoon of minced garlic

- 1 medium tomato (cut into 4 slices)

- 2 teaspoons of chopped fresh basil

- 1 cup of shredded mozzarella cheese

Kitchen Equipment:

- oven

- baking sheet

- aluminum foil

Directions:

1. Preheat the oven to broil.

2. Put aluminum foil in a baking sheet and set aside.

3. In a small bowl, toss the mushroom caps with the olive oil until well coated.

4. Use your fingertips to rub the oil in without breaking the mushrooms.

5. Arrange the mushrooms on the baking sheet gill-side down and broil the mushrooms until they are tender on the tops, about 2 minutes.

6. Flip the mushrooms over and broil 1 minute more.

7. Take the baking sheet out and spread the garlic over each mushroom, top each with a tomato slice, sprinkle with the basil, and top with the cheese.

8. Broil the mushrooms until the cheese is melted and bubbly, about 1 minute. Serve.

Nutrition:

Calories: 251 - **Fat:** 20g - **Protein:** 14g

4. SAUTÉED ASPARAGUS WITH WALNUTS

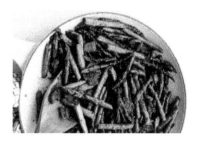

Dairy Free, Gluten Free, Vegetarian

Preparation Time: 10 minutes

Cooking Time: 5 minutes

Servings: 4

Ingredients:

- 1½ tablespoons of olive oil

- ¾ pound of asparagus (woody ends trimmed)

- Sea salt

- Freshly ground pepper

- ¼ cup of chopped walnuts

Kitchen Equipment:

- large skillet

Directions:

1. Situate a large skillet over medium-high heat and add the olive oil.

2. Sauté the asparagus until the spears are tender and lightly browned, about 5 minutes.

3. Season the asparagus with salt and pepper.

4. Remove the skillet from the heat and toss the asparagus with the walnuts. Serve.

Nutrition:

Calories: 124 - **Fat:** 12g - **Protein:** 3g

5. MUSHROOM OMELETTE

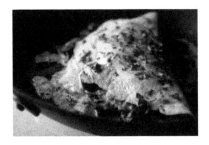

Gluten Free, Nut Free

Preparation Time: 10 minutes

Cooking Time: 15 minutes

Servings: 6

Ingredients:

- 2 tablespoons of olive oil

- 1 cup of sliced fresh mushrooms

- 1 cup of shredded spinach

- 6 bacon slices (cooked and chopped)

- 10 large eggs (beaten)

- ½ cup of crumbled goat cheese

- Sea salt

- Freshly ground black pepper

Kitchen Equipment:

- oven

- large ovenproof skillet

- spatula

Directions:

1. Preheat the oven to 350°F.

2. Situate a large ovenproof skillet over medium-high heat and pour the olive oil.

3. Sauté the mushrooms until lightly browned, about 3 minutes.

4. Add the spinach and bacon and sauté until the

greens are wilted, about 1 minute.

5. Add the eggs and cook, lifting the edges of the frittata with a spatula so uncooked egg flow underneath, for 3 to 4 minutes.

6. Top with the crumbled goat cheese and season lightly.

7. Bake until set and lightly browned, about 15 minutes.

8. Remove the frittata from the oven, and let it stand for 5 minutes.

9. Cut into 6 wedges and serve immediately.

Nutrition:

Calories: 316 - **Fat:** 27g - **Protein:** 16g

6. WALNUT HERB-CRUSTED GOAT CHEESE

Gluten Free, Vegetarian

Preparation Time: 10 minutes

Cooking Time: 0 minute

Servings: 4

Ingredients:

- 6 ounces of chopped walnuts

- 1 tablespoon of chopped oregano

- 1 tablespoon of chopped parsley

- 1 teaspoon of chopped fresh thyme

- ¼ teaspoon of freshly ground black pepper

- 1 (8-ounce) log of goat cheese

Kitchen Equipment:

- food processor

Directions:

1. Place the walnuts, oregano, parsley, thyme, and pepper in a food processor and pulse until finely chopped.

2. Pour the walnut mixture onto a plate and roll the goat cheese log in the nut mixture, pressing so the cheese is covered and the walnut mixture sticks to the log.

3. Wrap the cheese in plastic and store in the refrigerator for up to 1 week.

4. Slice and enjoy!

Nutrition: Calories: 304 - **Fat:** 28g - **Protein:** 12g

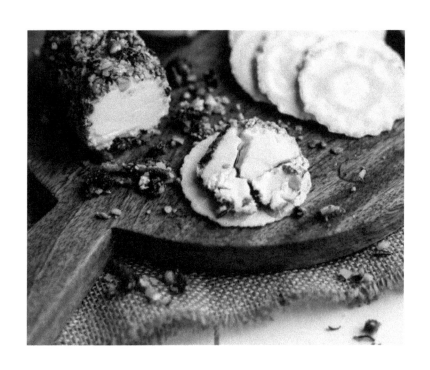

7. SMOKED SALMON AND LEEK SOUP

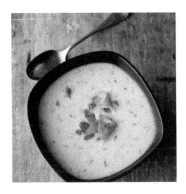

Preparation Time: 10 minutes

Cooking Time: 1 hour

Servings: 6

Ingredients:

- 2 tablespoons of extra-virgin olive oil

- ½ pound (227 g) of smoked salmon (roughly chopped)

- 1 fish stock cube

- 1 leek (finely chopped)

- 4 garlic cloves (crushed)

- 1 small onion (finely chopped)

- Salt (to taste)

- 1 cup of water

- 2 cups of heavy whipping cream

Kitchen Equipment:

- slow cooker

Directions:

1. Grease the insert of the slow cooker with 2 tablespoons of olive oil.

2. Combine the salmon, stock cube, leek, garlic, onion, salt, and water in the slow cooker.

3. Stir to mix well.

4. Seal the slow cooker lid on and cook on low heat for 2 hours, then mix in the cream and cook for 1 additional hour.

5. Take out the soup from the slow cooker to a large bowl.

6. Serve warm.

Nutrition: Calories: 219 - **Total fat:** 17.9g - **Fiber:** 0.5g

8. CHOCOLATE SEA SALT SMOOTHIE

Preparation Time: 5 minutes

Cooking Time: 0 minute

Servings: 2

Ingredients:

- 1 avocado (frozen or not)
- 2 cups of almond milk
- 1 tbsp. of tahini
- ¼ cup of cocoa powder
- 1 scoop of perfect Keto chocolate base

Kitchen Equipment:

- blender

Directions:

1. Incorporate all the ingredients in a high-speed blender and mix until you get a soft smoothie.

2. Add ice and enjoy!

Nutrition:

Calories: 235

Fat: 20g

Carbohydrates: 11.25

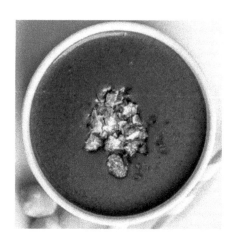

9. 5 INGREDIENT KETO SALAD

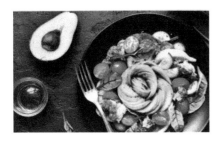

Preparation Time: 15 minutes

Cooking Time: 0 minute

Servings: 2

Ingredients:

- 2 boneless of chicken breasts with skin

- 1 large avocado (sliced)

- 3 slices of bacon

- 4 cups of mixed leafy greens of choice

- 2 tbsp. of dairy-free ranch dressing

- Salt and pepper to taste

- Duck fat for greasing

Kitchen Equipment:

- pan

- skillet

Directions:

3. Preheat the oven to 200 degrees Celsius or 400 degrees Fahrenheit.

4. Season the chicken with salt and pepper.

5. Grab a skillet and grease it with duck fat before cooking the chicken on the hot pan.

6. Keep the heat on high until you get a golden-brown skin surface.

7. Once done, you can cook the chicken in the oven for 10 to 15 minutes. You can also put the bacon in with the chicken to save on the cooking time. You can

also fry it in a pan, depending on your personal preferences.

8. After cooking, allow the chicken rest for a few minutes. Slice the avocado and the cooked chicken.

9. Start assembling your salad, adding together the leafy greens, crispy bacon, sliced chicken, and avocado.

10. Use 2 tablespoons of ranch dressing.

11. Mix together until all ingredients are thoroughly coated. Enjoy!

Nutrition:

Carbs: 3.1g - **Protein:** 38.7g - **Fat:** 43.8g

10. KETO BONE BROTH

Preparation Time: 10 minutes

Cooking Time: 80 minutes

Servings: 12

Ingredients:

- 3 Pastured Chicken Carcasses

- 10 cups of filtered water

- 2 tbsp. peppercorns

- 3 tsp. turmeric

- 1 tsp. salt

- 2 tbsp. apple cider vinegar

- 1 lemon

- 3 bay leaves

Kitchen Equipment:

- oven

- sheet pan

- slow cooker

- strainer

- mason jars

- large container

Directions:

1. Preheat the oven to 400 degrees Fahrenheit.

2. Put the bones on a sheet pan and slightly sprinkle with salt.

3. Roast the chicken for 45 minutes.

4. Transfer the cooked chicken to the slow cooker bowl.

5. Put in the peppercorns, apple cider vinegar, water, and bay leaves.

6. Cook on low heat for 23 hours.

7. When done, strain the bowl using a fine mesh sieve.

8. Discard the solid ingredients.

9. Divide the broth in mason jars, about 2 cups each container.

10. Put in 1 tsp. of turmeric for each day and 2 slices of lemon. If you're putting it in a large

container, just make sure to maintain the ration. Hence, if the large container has 4 cups worth of broth, you should put 2 teaspoons of turmeric and 4 slices of lemon inside.

11. Heat slowly and serve when needed

Nutrition:

Calories: 70 - **Fat:** 4g -
Carbohydrates: 1g

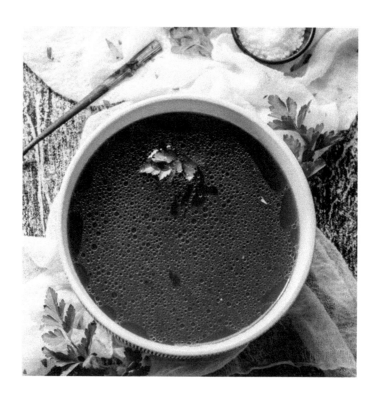

11. BEEF CABBAGE

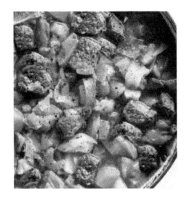

Preparation Time: 10 minutes

Cooking Time: 35 minutes

Servings: 8

Ingredients:

- 1-pound of scotch fillet steak (cut into 1-inch pieces)

- 1 large onion (chopped)

- 1 stalk of celery (chopped)

- 2 large carrots (diced)

- 1 small green cabbage chopped into bite-sized pieces

- 4 cloves garlic minced

- 6 cups of beef stock or broth

- 3 tbsp. of fresh chopped parsley

- 2 tbsp. of olive oil

- 2 tsp. of dried thyme

- 2 tsp. of dried rosemary

- 2 tsp. of onion or garlic powder

- Salt and freshly-cracked black pepper to taste

Kitchen Equipment:

- large pot

Directions:

1. Put oil in a large pot and apply medium heat.

2. Sear the beef on all sides until brown. They don't have to be cooked as they will be cooked later.

3. Put in the onions and cook them for 3 minutes

4. Put the celery and carrots.

5. Cook them while constantly stirring for 4 minutes.

6. Put in the cabbage and continue cooking until the cabbage softens up.

7. Put in the garlic until you get that very fragrant flavor.

8. Add the stock or broth. Follow it up with the dried herbs, parsley, and the onion or garlic powder. Remember that you're using low to medium heat all this time.

9. Mix well and bring it to a simmer. Cover the pot with a lid and leave it like that for 15 minutes.

10. Constantly check to see if the carrots are already cooked as these will take the longest.

11. When they're already soft, season the soup with salt and pepper to taste.

12. Serve hot and enjoy! Store this in the fridge for up to 3 days or even 2 months if you freeze them.

Nutrition:

Calories: 177

Carbohydrates: 4g

Protein: 12g

12. CHOCOLATE MUFFINS

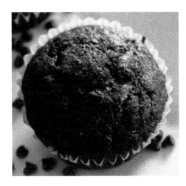

Preparation Time: 20 minutes

Cooking Time: 5 minutes

Servings: 6

Ingredients:

- ½ cup of coconut oil

- ½ cup of peanut butter

- Liquid stevia granulated sweetener (to your liking)

Kitchen Equipment:

- muffin tin or loaf pans

- stovetop or microwave

Directions:

1. Prepare the tin of choice with a spritz of oil.

2. Combine the oil and peanut butter together on the stovetop or microwave.

3. Melt and add the sweetener. Scoop into the tins or loaf pan and freeze.

4. You can serve with a drizzle of melted chocolate — but remember to count the carbs.

Nutrition:

Protein: 7g

Total Fats: 14g

Calories: 193

13. PEANUT BUTTER FUDGE

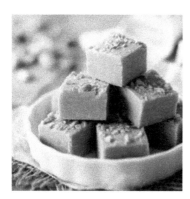

Preparation Time: 20 minutes

Cooking Time: 0 minutes

Servings: 20

Ingredients:

- 3 tbsp. of coconut oil

- 12 oz. of smooth peanut butter (Keto-friendly)

- 4 tbsp. of coconut cream

- 4 tbsp. of maple syrup

- Pinch of salt

Kitchen Equipment:

- parchment paper

- baking sheet

- stovetop

Directions:

1. Line a baking sheet with a layer of parchment paper.

2. Melt the syrup and coconut oil using the medium heat setting on the stovetop.

3. Stir in the salt, coconut cream, and peanut butter.

4. Pour the mixture into the prepared dish and chill in the fridge for at least one hour.

5. Slice into pieces and store or serve.

Nutrition: Protein: 4g - **Total Fats:** 11g - **Calories:** 135

14. PEANUT BUTTER MOUSSE

Preparation Time: 20 minutes

Cooking Time: 0 minute

Servings: 3

Ingredients:

- ½ cup of heavy whipping cream

- 4 oz. of room temp cream cheese

- ¼ cup of powdered Swerve Sweetener

- ¼ cup of sugar-free natural peanut butter

- ½ tsp. of vanilla extract

Kitchen Equipment:

- medium bowl

- container

Directions:

1. In a medium bowl, beat the cream until it creates stiff peaks. Set aside for now.

2. In another mixing container, beat the cream cheese, sweetener, peanut butter, and vanilla. Add a pinch of salt if the peanut butter is unsalted.

3. Mix until creamy smooth. If your mixture is overly thick, add about two tablespoons of heavy cream to lighten it and continue mixing.

4. Gently fold in the whipped cream. Spoon or use a piping tool to add it into dessert glasses.

5. Drizzle using a portion of low-carb chocolate sauce or other toppings, as desired. (Be sure to

count the additional
carbs.)

Nutrition: **Calories:** 301 -
Protein: 5.9g - **Total Fats:**
26.5g

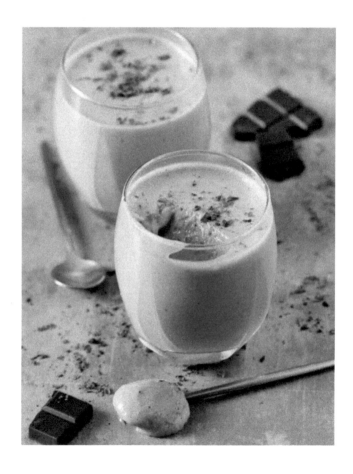

15. CHOCOLATE PEANUT BUTTER CUPS

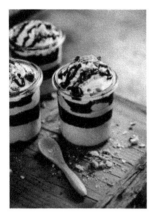

Preparation Time: 15 minutes

Cooking Time: 3 minutes

Servings: 12

Ingredients:

- 1 oz. of roasted peanuts (chopped and salted)

- 1 cup of coconut oil

- ¼ tsp. of kosher salt

- ½ cup of natural peanut butter

- ¼ tsp. of vanilla extract

- 2 tbsp. of heavy cream

- 1 tsp. of liquid stevia

- 1 tbsp. of cocoa powder

Kitchen Equipment:

- stove

- saucepan

- 12 silicon molds

- baking sheet

Directions:

1. You'll need your stove at low heat for this recipe.

2. Place a saucepan on the heat and add coconut oil.

3. After about 5 minutes, add peanut butter, salt, heavy cream, cocoa powder, vanilla extract, and liquid stevia to the pan.

4. Stir till the peanut butter melts.

5. Get 12 silicone muffin molds and pour the peanut butter mixture in it.

6. Add the salted peanuts on top.

7. Transfer the muffin molds to a baking sheet and place the pan in your freezer.

8. Let it stay in the freezer for an hour, and then unmold the cups.

9. Place the chocolate peanut cups in any airtight container.

Nutrition:

Calories: 246 - **Carbs:** 3.3g - **Protein:** 3.4g

16. PEANUT BUTTER COOKIES

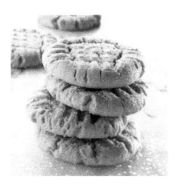

Preparation Time: 10 minutes

Cooking Time: 15 minutes

Servings: 12

Ingredients:

- 1 tsp. of vanilla extract, sugar-free

- 1 cup of peanut butter

- 1 egg

- ½ cup of natural sweetener (low-calorie)

Kitchen Equipment:

- oven

- baking sheet

- wire rack

Directions:

1. Prepare the oven to 350 degrees Fahrenheit.

2. Follow that by preparing a baking sheet. Line the sheet using parchment paper.

3. Into a bowl, add peanut butter, vanilla extract, sweetener, and egg. Mix these ingredients well until you are left with dough.

4. Using your hands, mold the dough into balls. These balls should be no more than 1 inch in size. Place them on the baking sheet you had prepared and flatten them with a fork. You'll probably love the pattern that forms on the flattened dough.

5. Put the baking sheet in the oven and let the cookies bake for 15 minutes. Afterwards, take

the pan out of the oven and just let it sit.

6. After a minute of cooling, it should be safe for you to place on a wire rack to cool even further.

Nutrition: **Calories:** 133 - **Protein:** 5.9g - **Fat:** 11.2g

17. CHOCOLATE FAT BOMB

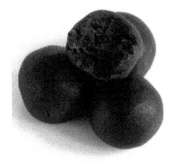

Preparation Time: 10 minutes

Cooking Time: 0 minute

Servings: 10

Ingredients:

- 1.4 oz. pack of instant chocolate pudding mix (sugar free)

- 8 oz. pack of cream cheese (softened)

- Coconut oil to your preferred taste (suggested: ¾ cup)

Kitchen Equipment:

- medium bowl

- electric mixer

- molds

- plastic wraps

Directions:

1. Into a medium bowl, add the chocolate pudding mix, cream cheese, and coconut oil.

2. Use an electric mixer to mix these ingredients until they are smooth.

3. Place this mixture into a mold to form into mounds.

4. Cover these mounds with plastic wraps and keep in your refrigerator for about 30 minutes. They should harden during this time.

Nutrition:

Calories: 231

Protein: 1.9g

Fat: 24.3g

18. KETO MATCHA MINT BARS

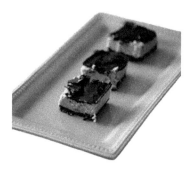

Preparation Time: 15 minutes

Cooking Time: 0 minute

Servings: 12

Ingredients:

- 6 drops of stevia
- 1 cup of almond flour (blanched)
- ¼ tsp. of peppermint extract
- 3 tbsp. of melted butter
- 3 tbsp. of cocoa powder
- Separate 1 tbsp. of cocoa powder (unsweetened)
- 3 tbsp. of warmed coconut oil
- 1 tbsp. of stevia powder
- 1 tsp. of vanilla extract
- 1 cup of softened coconut butter
- Separate 1 tsp. of peppermint extract
- 2 small ripe avocados
- 1 tbsp. of Matcha (green tea powder)
- Separate 3 tbsp. of stevia powder

Kitchen Equipment:

- 8x8-inch baking pan
- parchment paper
- medium bowl

Directions:

1. Before anything, prepare an 8x8" baking pan. Do this by lining the pan with parchment paper.

2. Into a medium bowl, add almond flour, stevia powder, cocoa powder, and butter. Mix these ingredients properly, and then pour the mixture into the prepared pan.

3. Press down on it till a crust is formed.

4. Transfer the baking pan in the freezer for 15 minutes.

5. It's time to prepare the filling. Again, you'll need a medium bowl. Add 3 tbsp. of stevia powder, coconut butter, vanilla extract, Matcha, avocados, and 1 tsp. of peppermint extract.

6. Use an electric mixer to mix these ingredients.

7. Take the baking pan out of the freezer and pour this Matcha mixture on the crust.

8. Return the pan to the freezer.

9. Finally, combine liquid stevia, coconut oil, 1 tbsp. of cocoa powder, and 1 tsp. of peppermint extract. Make sure you mix these ingredients well before pouring them over the bars. You can leave them in the refrigerator throughout the night or for just 30 minutes.

Nutrition:

Calories: 276

Protein: 4.3g

Fat: 26.1g

19. CHICKEN NUGGETS WITH SWEET POTATO CRUSTING

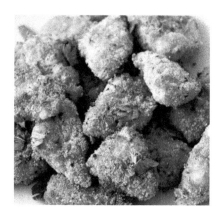

Preparation Time: 10 minutes

Cooking Time: 30 minutes

Servings: 4

Ingredients:

- 1 cup of sweet potato chips
- ¼ cup of flour
- 1 tsp. of salt
- ½ tsp. of ground pepper (ground)
- ¼ tsp. of baking powder
- 1 tbsp. of cornstarch
- 1 pound of chicken tenderloins (cut in pieces of half-inch)
- Oil (to fry)

Kitchen Equipment:

- large skillet
- food processor

Directions:

1. Heat the oil in a large skillet.
2. Add flour, chips, salt, baking powder, and pepper in a food processor.
3. Pulse the ingredients for making a ground mixture.
4. Toss the chicken pieces in cornstarch.
5. Shake off excess cornstarch.
6. Toss in the chip mixture.
7. Press the chicken pieces gently for coating.

8. Fry the chicken nuggets for three minutes.

9. Serve hot.

Nutrition: **Calories:** 305.6 - **Protein:** 26.6g - **Fat:** 18.9g

20. TACO EGG MUFFINS

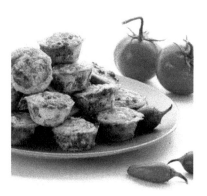

Preparation Time: 10 minutes

Cooking Time: 30 minutes

Servings: 8

Ingredients:

- ½ lb. of ground beef, grass-fed

- 1 ½ tbsp. of taco seasoning

- 1 tbsp. of salted butter (melted)

- 3 eggs (organic)

- 3 oz. of Mexican cheese blend (shredded and full-fat)

- ½ cup of tomato salsa (organic)

Kitchen Equipment:

- oven

- skillet pan

- parchment paper

- silicone muffin cups

Directions:

1. Preheat oven at 350 degrees F.

2. Meanwhile, place a skillet pan over medium heat, grease with oil and when hot, mix in ground beef and cook for 7 minutes or more until almost cooked.

3. Season beef with the taco seasoning and cook for 3 to 5 minutes or until cooked through, and then remove the pan from heat.

4. Break eggs in a bowl, whisk until beaten, then add cooked taco beef along with 2 ounces of

Mexican cheese and whisk until well combined.

5. Take a 32 cups muffin pan, or parchment-lined silicone muffin cups, grease each cup with melted butter, then evenly fill with taco beef mixture and top with remaining cheese.

6. Situate muffin pan into the oven and bake for 20 minutes or until muffins are cooked through, and the top is nicely golden brown.

7. When done, let muffins cool in the pan for 10 minutes, then take them out and cool on a wire rack.

8. Serve muffins with salsa.

Nutrition: **Calories:** 329 - **Fat:** 22.15g - **Protein:** 25.2g

21. CHICKEN, BACON, AVOCADO CAESAR SALAD

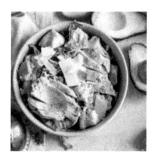

Preparation Time: 10 minutes

Cooking Time: 0 minute

Servings: 4

Ingredients:

- 1 chicken breast (pre-cooked or grilled, sliced into small bite sized slices)

- 1 avocado (ripe, slice into approximately 1" slices)

- Creamy Caesar dressing (approximately 3 tablespoons per salad)

- 1 cup of bacon (pre-cooked, crumbled)

Kitchen Equipment:

- large-sized bowl.

Directions:

1. Combine the chicken breast with avocado slices and crumbled bacon between two large sized bowls.

2. Top with a spoonful of the Creamy Caesar dressing; lightly toss the ingredients.

3. Serve immediately and enjoy.

Nutrition:

Calories: 322

Total Fat: 30g

Total Carbohydrates: 5g

22. COCONUT MACADAMIA BARS

Preparation Time: 15 minutes

Cooking Time: 0 minute

Servings: 6

Ingredients:

- ½ cup of macadamia nuts

- 6 tablespoons of unsweetened coconut (shredded)

- ½ cup of almond butter

- 20 drops of stevia drops (preferably sweet leaf)

- ¼ cup of coconut oil

Kitchen Equipment:

- food processor

- large-sized mixing bowl

- 9x9-inch baking dish

- parchment paper

Directions:

1. Crush the macadamia nuts using hands or in a food processor.

2. Combine coconut oil with the shredded coconut and almond butter in a large-sized mixing bowl.

3. Add the stevia drops and chopped macadamia nuts.

4. Thoroughly mix and pour the prepared batter into a 9x9" baking dish lined with parchment paper.

5. Refrigerate for overnight; slice into desired pieces. Serve and enjoy.

Nutrition: **Calories:** 324 - **Total Fat:** 32g - **Total Carbohydrates:** 5g

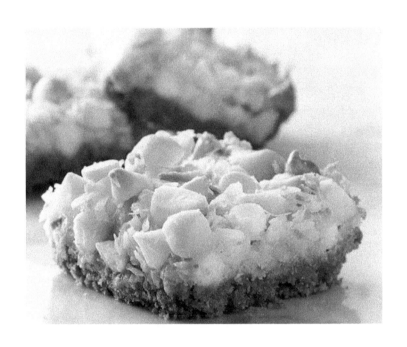

23. MACADAMIA CHOCOLATE FAT BOMB

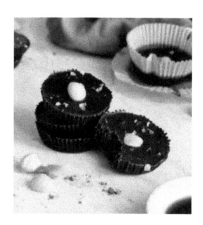

Preparation Time: 15 minutes

Cooking Time: 0 minute

Servings: 6

Ingredients:

- 2 oz. of cocoa butter

- 4 oz. of macadamias (chopped)

- 2 tablespoons of Swerve

- ¼ cup of coconut oil or heavy cream

- 2 tablespoons of cocoa powder (unsweetened)

Kitchen Equipment:

- large saucepan

- small saucepan

- paper candy cups or molds

Directions:

1. Pour a half full of boiling water onto a large sauce pan.

2. Place a small sized saucepan over the large sauce pan with the boiling water and melt the cocoa butter in it.

3. Once melted, incorporate the cocoa powder and then add the Swerve; mix well until the entire ingredients are completely melted and well blended.

4. Add in the macadamias; give everything a good stir.

5. Now, add the cream or coconut oil; mix well (bringing it to the temperature again).

6. Pour the prepared mixture into paper candy cups or molds; filling them evenly.

7. Let cool for a couple of minutes at room temperature and then place them in a refrigerator.

8. Let chill until harden. Serve and enjoy.

Nutrition: Calories: 267 - **Total Fat:** 28g - **Total Carbohydrates:** 3g

24. KETO LEMON BREAKFAST FAT BOMBS

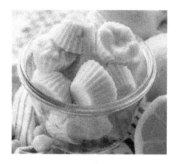

25.

Preparation Time: 10 minutes + 50 minutes of refrigeration

Cooking Time: 0 minute

Servings: 6

Ingredients:

- 10 to 15 drops of Stevia extract

- 1 tablespoon of lemon extract or lemon zest (organic)

- 1 pack of coconut butter or creamed coconut (approximately 3.5 oz.), softened

- 1 oz. of extra-virgin coconut oil, softened (approximately 1/8 cup)

- A pinch of Himalayan pink salt or sea salt

Kitchen Equipment:

- large-sized mixing bowls

- silicon candy mold or mini muffin paper cup

- large-sized tray

Directions:

1. Zest the lemons and ensure that the coconut oil and coconut butter are at room temperature and softened.

2. Combine the entire ingredients together in a large-sized mixing bowl and ensure the stevia and lemon zest are evenly distributed.

3. Fill each silicone candy mold or mini muffin paper cup with approximately 1

tablespoon of the prepared coconut mixture and place them on a large-sized tray.

4. Place the tray inside the fridge and let chill until solid, for 40 to 50 minutes.

5. Keep refrigerated until ready to serve. Serve and enjoy.

Nutrition: **Calories:** 184 - **Total Fat:** 20g - **Total Carbohydrates:** 0.2g

26. SPICY CHICKEN THIGHS

Preparation Time: 10 minutes

Cooking Time: 15 minutes

Servings: 4

Ingredients:

- 1-pound of chicken thighs (boneless)

- A small handful of fresh cilantros (for garnish)

- ½ tablespoon of chili powder

- Lime wedges (fresh for serving)

- ½ tablespoon of extra-virgin olive oil (organic)

- Fresh ground pepper and sea salt to taste

Kitchen Equipment:

- oven

- sheet pan

Directions:

1. Preheat your oven to 375°F.

2. Place the chicken thighs on a sheet pan, and drizzle with the olive oil; turn several times until evenly coated with the oil.

3. Now, rub the chicken pieces with chili powder, pepper, and salt.

4. Roast the chicken thighs for 12 to 15 minutes, until cooked through.

5. Sprinkle with fresh cilantro; serve immediately with some lime wedges and enjoy.

Nutrition: Calories: 246 - **Total Fat:** 13g - **Total Carbohydrates:** 2.3g

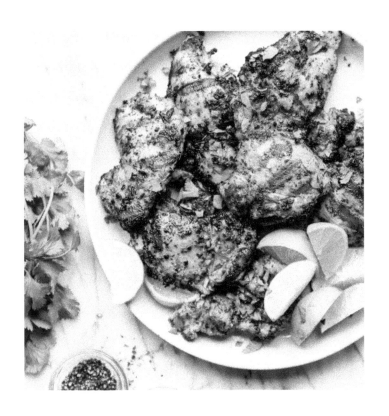

27. CHICKEN QUESADILLAS

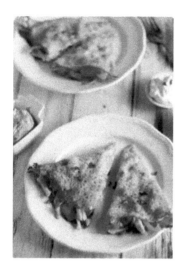

Preparation Time: 10 minutes

Cooking Time: 15 minutes

Servings: 2

Ingredients:

- 1½ cups of mozzarella cheese (shredded)

- 1½ cups of cheddar cheese (shredded)

- 1 cup of chicken (cooked and shredded)

- 1 bell pepper (sliced)

- ¼ cup of tomato (diced)

- 1/8 cup of green onion

- 1 tbsp. of extra-virgin olive oil

Kitchen Equipment:

- oven

Directions:

1. Preheat the oven to 400°F. Use parchment paper to cover a pizza pan.

2. Combine your cheeses and bake the cheese shell for about 5 minutes.

3. Put the chicken on one half of the cheese shell.

4. Add peppers, tomatoes, green onion and fold your shell in half over the fillings.

5. Return your folded cheese shell to the oven again for 4–5 minutes.

Nutrition: **Carbohydrates:** 6.1g - **Fat:** 40.5g - **Protein:** 52,7g

28. SHRIMP LETTUCE WRAPS WITH BUFFALO SAUCE

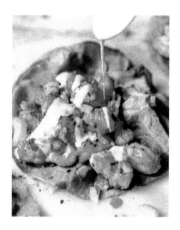

Preparation Time: 15 minutes

Cooking Time: 20 minutes

Servings: 4

Ingredients:

- 1 egg (beaten)
- 3 tbsp. of butter
- 16 oz. of shrimp (peeled, deveined, with tails removed)
- ¾ cup of almond flour
- ¼ cup of hot sauce (like Frank's)
- 1 tsp. of extra-virgin olive oil
- Kosher salt
- Black pepper
- Garlic
- 1 head romaine lettuce (leaves parted, for serving)
- ½ red onion (chopped)
- Celery (finely sliced)
- ½ blue cheese (cut into pieces)

Kitchen Equipment:

- saucepan
- large frying pan

Directions:

1. To make the Buffalo sauce, melt the butter in a saucepan, add the garlic and cook this mixture for 1 minute.

2. Pour hot sauce into the saucepan and whisk to combine. Set aside.

3. In one bowl, crack one egg, add salt and pepper and mix.

4. In another bowl, put the almond flour, add salt and pepper and also combine.

5. Dip each shrimp into the egg mixture first and then into the almond one.

6. Take a large frying pan. Heat the oil and cook your shrimp for about 2 minutes per side.

7. Add Buffalo sauce.

8. Serve in lettuce leaves. Top your shrimp with red onion, blue cheese, and celery.

Nutrition: Carbohydrates: 8g - **Fat:** 54g - **Protein:** 33g

29. WRAPPED BACON CHEESEBURGER

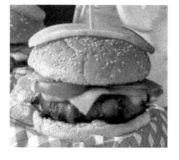

Preparation Time: 15 minutes

Cooking Time: 8 minutes

Servings: 4

Ingredients:

- 7 oz. of bacon

- 1½ pounds of ground beef

- ½ tsp. of salt

- ¼ tsp. of pepper

- 4 oz. of cheese (shredded)

- 1 head iceberg or romaine lettuce (leaves parted and washed)

- 1 tomato (sliced)

- ¼ pickled cucumber (finely sliced)

Kitchen Equipment:

- frying pan

Directions:

1. Cook the bacon and set aside.

2. In a separate bowl, combine ground beef, salt, and pepper. Divide the mixture into 4 sections, create balls and press each one slightly to form a patty.

3. Put your patties into a frying pan and cook for about 4 minutes on each side.

4. Top each cooked patty with a slice of cheese, several pieces of bacon, and pickled cucumber.

5. Add a bit of tomato.

6. Wrap each burger in a big lettuce leaf.

Nutrition: **Carbohydrates:** 5g - **Protein:** 48g - **Calories:** 684

30. FATTY BURGER BOMBS

Preparation Time: 15 minutes

Cooking Time: 15 minutes

Servings: 20

Ingredients:

- 1-pound of ground beef

- ½ tsp. of garlic powder

- Kosher salt and black pepper

- 1 oz. of cold butter (cut into 20 pieces)

- ½ block of cheddar cheese (cut into 20 pieces)

Kitchen Equipment:

- oven

- mini muffin tin

Directions:

1. Preheat the oven to 375°F.

2. In a separate bowl, the mix ground beef, garlic powder, salt, and pepper.

3. Use a mini muffin tin to form your bombs.

4. Put about 1 tbsp. of beef into each muffin tin cup. Make sure that you completely cover the bottom.

5. Add a piece of butter on top and put 1 tbsp. of beef over the butter.

6. Place a piece of cheese on the top and put the remaining beef over the cheese.

7. Bake your bombs for about 15 minutes.

Nutrition: Fat: 7g - **Protein:** 5g - **Calories:** 80

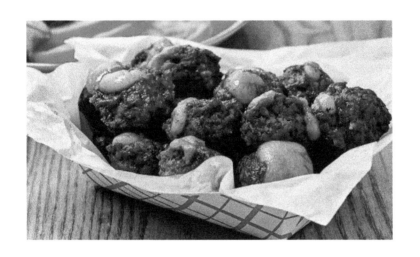

31. AVOCADO TACO

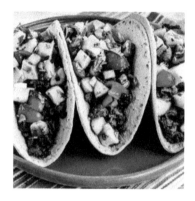

Preparation Time: 10 minutes

Cooking Time: 15 minutes

Servings: 6

Ingredients:

- 1-pound of ground beef
- 3 avocados (halved)
- 1 tbsp. of chili powder
- ½ tsp. of salt
- ¾ tsp. of cumin
- ½ tsp. of oregano (dried)
- ¼ tsp. of garlic powder
- ¼ tsp. of onion powder
- 8 tbsp. of tomato sauce
- 1 cup of cheddar cheese (shredded)
- ¼ cup of cherry tomatoes (sliced)
- ¼ cup of lettuce (shredded)
- ½ cup of sour cream

Kitchen Equipment:

- saucepan

Directions:

1. Pit halved avocados.
2. Set aside.
3. Place the ground beef into a saucepan and cook over medium heat until it is browned.
4. Add the seasoning and tomato sauce.
5. Stir well and cook for about 4 minutes.
6. Load each avocado half with the beef.
7. Top with shredded cheese and lettuce,

tomato slices, and sour cream.

Nutrition: Fat 22g - **Protein** 18g - **Calories** 278

32. CREAMY MUSHROOMS WITH GARLIC AND THYME

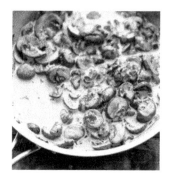

Preparation Time: 5 minutes

Cooking Time: 15 minutes

Servings: 4

Ingredients:

- 4 tbsp. of unsalted butter

- ½ cup of onion (chopped)

- 1-pound of button mushrooms

- 2 tsp. of garlic (diced)

- 1 tbs. of fresh thyme

- 1 tbsp. parsley (chopped)

- ½ tsp. of salt

- ¼ tsp. of black pepper

Kitchen Equipment:

- sauté pan

Directions:

1. Melt the butter in a pan.

2. Place the mushrooms into the pan.

3. Add salt and pepper.

4. Cook the mushroom mix for about 5 minutes until they're browned on both sides.

5. Add the garlic and thyme.

6. Additionally, sauté the mushrooms for 1-2 minutes.

7. Top them with parsley.

Nutrition: Fat: 8g - **Protein:** 3g - **Calories:** 99

33. ONE SHEET FAJITAS

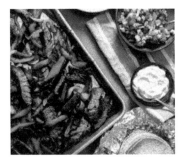

Preparation Time: 5 minutes

Cooking Time: 20 minutes

Servings: 6

Ingredients:

- 1 lb. of chicken breast
- 2 tbsp. of fajita seasoning
- ¼ cup of cilantro
- 1 sliced of onion
- 1 sliced of red bell pepper
- 1 sliced of green bell pepper
- 3 tbsp. of olive Oil
- A dash salt
- 2 tbsp. of lime juice

Kitchen Equipment:

- pan
- stove
- oven
- baking sheet

Directions:

1. Preheat the oven to 400°F. As this warms up, you can also get out the one baking sheet.

2. Throw all of the ingredients from above into a mixing bowl and season with the pepper, salt, and the lime juice.

3. Once this is set, spread the items across your baking sheet as evenly as possible.

4. Pop it into the stove for 20 minutes. By the end of this time, the chicken should be cooked through. If you like everything a little crispy, you can go ahead and broil the ingredients for an additional two minutes.

5. When your meal is set, take it out from the stove and allow it to chill for two minutes.

6. As a final touch, season with some fresh cilantro and enjoy your Keto-friendly fajitas!

Nutrition: Fats: 10g - **Carbs:** 4g - **Proteins:** 25g

34. SPICY KETO CHICKEN WINGS

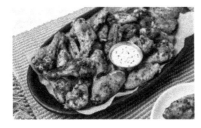

Preparation Time: 10 minutes

Cooking Time: 60 minutes

Servings: 4

Ingredients:

- 2 lb. of chicken wings
- 1 tsp. of Cajun spice
- 2 tsp. of smoked paprika
- ½ tsp. of turmeric
- A dash of salt
- 2 tsp. of baking powder
- A dash of pepper

Kitchen Equipment:

- mixing bowl
- wire rack
- baking tray
- baking sheet
- stove

Directions:

1. Prepare the stove to 400°F and take some time to dry your chicken wings with a paper towel to remove any excess moisture and get you some nice, crispy wings!

2. When you are all set, take out a mixing bowl and place all of the seasonings along with the baking powder.

3. Once these are set, throw the chicken wings in and coat evenly. If you have one, you'll want to place the wings on a wire rack that is placed over your baking tray. If not, you can just lay them across the baking sheet.

4. Pop them into the stove for thirty minutes. By the end of this time, the tops of the wings should be crispy. If they are,

take them out from the oven and flip them so that you can bake the other side. You will want to cook these for an additional thirty minutes.

5. Take the tray from the oven and allow cooling slightly before serving up your spiced Keto wings. For additional flavor, serve with any of your favorite, Keto-friendly dipping sauce.

Nutrition: **Fats:** 7g - **Carbs:** 1g - **Proteins:** 60g

35. GROUND BEEF BOWL

Preparation Time: 10 minutes

Cooking Time: 20 minutes

Servings: 4

Ingredients:

For Cauliflower Rice:

- 1 lb. of cauliflower (riced)

- ½ tsp. of sea salt

- 1/8 tsp. of ground black pepper

- 1 tbsp. of avocado oil

For the Beef:

- 1 lb. of beef (grass-fed)

- ½ tsp. of sea salt

- 2 tbsp. of minced garlic

- ¼ cup of coconut aminos

- ¼ tsp. of ground ginger

- ¼ tsp. of crushed red pepper flakes

- 1 tbsp. of avocado oil

- 2 tsp. of sesame oil

- ¼ cup of beef broth (grass-fed)

For the Garnish:

- ¼ cup of sliced green onions

- 1 tsp. of sesame seeds

Kitchen Equipment:

- large skillet pan

- microwave

Directions:

1. Prepare cauliflower rice and for this, take a large skillet pan, place it over medium-high heat, add oil and when hot, add cauliflower rice, season with salt and black pepper and cook for 5 minutes or until thoroughly cooked.

2. Then remove the pan from the heat, transfer to

65

a bowl, and set aside until required.

3. Prepare the sauce and for this, whisk together ginger, coconut aminos, red pepper flakes, sesame oil, and beef broth until combined, and set aside until required.

4. Return skillet pan over medium-high heat, add avocado oil and when hot, add beef, season with salt and cook for 10 minutes or until light brown.

5. Make the well in the pan, add garlic in it, and let it cook for 1 minute or until sauté, then mix it into the beef and pour in the prepared sauce.

6. Stir well and let beef simmer for 4 minutes or until sauce is thickened and not much liquid is left in the pan.

7. Remove pan from the heat and let beef cool completely.

8. Portion out the beef and cauliflower into four glass meal prep containers, garnish with green onion and sesame seeds, then seal the lid and stock in the freezing for up to 2 months.

9. When ready to serve, reheat the beef and cauliflower in its glass vial in the microwave until cook.

Nutrition:

Calories: 513 - **Fat:** 36g - **Protein:** 35g

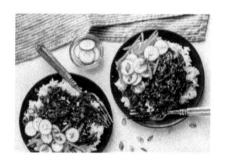

36. AVOCADO DIP

Preparation Time: 10 minutes

Cooking Time: 0 minute

Servings: 4

Ingredients:

- 2 Organic avocados (pitted)

- 1/3 medium organic red onion (peeled and sliced)

- 1 medium organic jalapeño (deseeded and diced)

- ½ tsp. of salt

- ½ tsp. of ground pepper

- 2 tbsp. of tomato salsa (organic)

- 1 tbsp. of lime juice (organic)

- ½ bunch of organic cilantros

Kitchen Equipment:

- bowl

Directions:

1. Cut each avocado into half, remove its pit and slice its flesh horizontally and vertically.

2. Take out the flesh of the avocado, place it in a bowl and add onion, jalapeno, and lime juice then stir until well mixed.

3. Season with salt and black pepper, add salsa and stir with a fork until avocado is mash to desired consistency. Fold in cilantro and serve.

Nutrition:

Calories: 16.5 - **Fat:** 1.4g - **Protein:** 0.23g

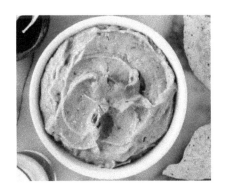

37. CHICKEN STUFFED CASSEROLE

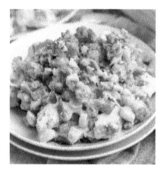

Preparation Time: 19 minutes

Cooking Time: 29 minutes

Servings: 4

Ingredients:

- 6 Tortilla Factory low-carb whole wheat tortillas (torn into small pieces)

- 1 ½ cups of hand-shredded cheese (Mexican)

- 1 beaten egg

- 1 cup of milk

- 2 cups of cooked chicken (shredded)

- 1 can of ro-tel

- ½ cup of salsa Verde

Kitchen Equipment:

- 8x8 glass baking dish

- oven

- freezer containers

Directions:

1. Brush an 8 x 8 glass baking dish with margarine.

2. Heat the oven to 375 degrees.

3. Combine everything, but reserve ½ cup of 8 x 8 glass baking tray with oil.

4. Heat the oven to 375 degrees. Combine everything, but reserve ½ cup of the cheese.

5. Bake it for 29 minutes. Take it out of the stove

and add ½ cup of cheese.

6. Broil for about 2 minutes to fade the cheese. Let the casserole cool.

7. Slice into 6 strips and place in freezer containers, (1 cup with a lid). Freeze.

8. Microwave for cool.

9. Slice into 6 slices and arrange in freezer containers, (1 cup with a lid). Freeze.

10. Microwave for 2 minutes to serve.

11. Top with sour cream, if desired.

Nutrition: **Calories:** 265 - **Total Fat:** 16g - **Protein:** 20g

38. STEAK SALAD WITH ASIAN SPICE

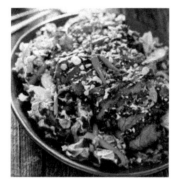

Preparation Time: 4 minutes

Cooking Time: 4 minutes

Servings: 2

Ingredients:

- 2 tablespoon of sriracha sauce

- 1 tablespoon of garlic (minced)

- 1 tablespoon of ginger (fresh, grated)

- 1 bell pepper, yellow (cut into thin strips)

- 1 bell pepper, red (cut into thin strips)

- 1 tablespoon of sesame oil (garlic)

- 1 Splenda of packet

- ½ tablespoon of curry powder

- ½ tablespoon rice wine vinegar

- 8 oz. of beef sirloin (cut into strips)

- 2 cups of baby spinach (stemmed)

- ½ head of butter lettuce (torn or chopped into bite-sized pieces)

Kitchen Equipment:

- zip-lock bag

Directions:

1. Place the garlic, sriracha sauce, 1 tablespoon of sesame oil, rice wine marinade, and Splenda into a bowl and combine well.

2. Pour half of this mix into a vigor-lock bag.

3. Add the steak to marinade while you are preparing the salad.

4. Assemble the brightly colored salad by layering in two bowls.

5. Place the baby spinach into the bottom of the bowl. Place the butter lettuce next.

6. Mix the two peppers and place on top.

7. Remove the steak from the marinade and discard the liquid and bag.

8. Heat the sesame oil and rapidly stir fry the steak until desired doneness, it should have about 3 minutes.

9. Situate the steak on top of the salad.

10. Drizzle with the remaining dressing (another field of marinade mix).

11. Sprinkle the sriracha sauce across the potato salad.

12. Combine the salad. Place the sriracha sauce into a small closed container.

13. Slice the steak and freeze in a zip-lock bag with container. Slice the steak and freeze in a zip-lock bag with the bathe.

14. To prepare, mix the ingredients like. To qualify, mix the ingredients like the initial

15. Directions: Stir fry the pickled beef for 4 minutes to take into consideration the beef is frozen.

Nutrition:

Calories: 350

Total Fat: 23g

Protein: 28g

39. STIR FRY CHICKEN

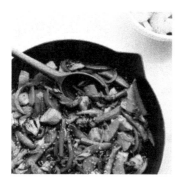

Preparation Time: 9 minutes

Cooking Time: 14 minutes

Servings: 4

Ingredients:

- 1/2 cup of sliced onion

- 2 tablespoon of oil (sesame garlic flavored)

- 4 cups of shredded bok-choy

- 1 cup of sugar snap peas

- 1 cup of fresh bean sprouts

- 3 stalks of celery (chopped)

- 1 1/2 tablespoon of minced garlic

- 1 packet of splenda

- 1 cup of broth, chicken

- 2 tablespoon of soy sauce

- 1 tablespoon of ginger (freshly minced)

- 1 tablespoon of cornstarch

- 4 boneless of chicken breasts (cooked/sliced thinly)

Kitchen Equipment:

- skillet pan

Directions:

1. Place the bok-choy, peas, celery in a skillet with 1 tbsp. of garlic oil.

2. Stir fry until bok-choy is diminished to liking.

3. Add remaining ingredients except for the cornstarch.

4. If too narrow, stir cornstarch into ½ cup lukewarm water when smooth flow into skillet.

5. Bring cornstarch and chow mien to a one-minute boil. Turn off the heat source.

6. Stir sauce then wait for 4 minutes to serve, after the chow mien has thickened.

7. Freeze in covered containers.

8. Heat for 2 minutes in the microwave before serving.

Nutrition: **Calories:** 369 - **Total Fat:** 18g - **Protein:** 42g

40. MEXICAN SHREDDED BEEF

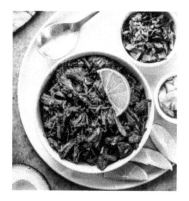

Preparation Time: 10 minutes

Cooking Time: 75 minutes

Servings: 8

Ingredients:

- 3 ½ lbs. of beef short ribs (grass-fed)
- 2 tbsp. of minced garlic
- 2 tsp. of ground turmeric
- 1 tsp. of salt
- ½ tsp. of ground black pepper
- 2 tsp. of ground cumin
- 2 tsp. of ground coriander
- 1 tsp. of chipotle powder
- ½ cup of water
- 1 cup of cilantro stems (chopped)

Kitchen Equipment:

- slow cooker
- small saucepan
- microwave

Directions:

1. Place salt in a small bowl, add black pepper, cumin, coriander, chipotle powder and stir until mixed.

2. Place ribs into the slow cooker, sprinkle well with the prepared spice mix and then top with minced garlic and cilantro stems.

3. Switch on the slow cooker, pour in water, then cover with the lid

and cook for 6 to 7 hours over low heat setting or until tender.

4. Fill the sauce into a small saucepan and cook for 10 to 15 minutes or until reduced by half.

5. Return the sauce into the slow cooker, pull apart the meat and toss until well mixed.

6. Portion out beef into eight glass meal prep containers, then wrap the lid and keep in the refrigerator for up to 5 days.

7. Upon serving, reheat the beef in its glass container in the microwave.

Nutrition: **Calories:** 656 - **Fat:** 48.5g - **Protein:** 50.2g

41. VEGETARIAN KETO COBB

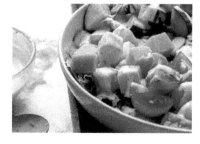

Preparation Time: 10 minutes

Cooking Time: 0 minute

Servings: 3

Ingredients:

- 3 large hard-boiled eggs (sliced)

- 4 ounces of cheddar cheese (cubed)

- 2 tbsp. of sour cream

- 2 tbsp. of mayonnaise

- ½ tsp. of garlic powder

- ½ tsp. of onion powder

- 1 tsp. of dried parsley

- 1 tbsp. of milk

- 1 tbsp. of Dijon mustard

- 3 cups of romaine lettuce (torn)

- 1 cup of cucumber (diced)

- ½ cup of cherry tomatoes (halved)

Kitchen Equipment:

- bowl

Directions:

1. The dressing is a combination of the source cream, mayonnaise, and dried herbs.

2. Mix them well together until full combined.

3. Add one tablespoon of milk into the mix until you get the thickness you want.

4. Layer in the salad, adding all the ingredients that

are not part of the dressing recipe.

5. Put the mustard on the center of the salad.

6. Drizzle with your dressing and enjoy!

7. Each serving should have just 2 tablespoons of dressing.

Nutrition: **Calories:** 330 - **Fat:** 26.32g - **Protein:** 16.82g

42. CHOCO MUG BROWNIE

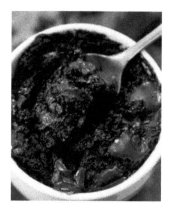

Preparation Time: 10 minutes

Cooking Time: 30 seconds

Servings: 1

Ingredients:

- 1 tbsp. of cocoa powder

- ½ tsp. of baking powder

- 1 scoop of chocolate protein powder

- ¼ cup of almond milk

Kitchen Equipment:

- mug

Directions:

1. Prepare a mug using the protein powder, cocoa, and baking powder.

2. Transfer the milk into the mug and stir.

3. Microwave for about 30 seconds and serve.

Nutrition:

Protein Counts: 12.4g

Total Fats: 15.8g

Calories: 207

43. CHOCOLATE PEANUT BUTTER CUPS

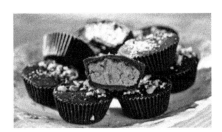

Preparation Time: 60 minutes

Cooking Time: 5 minutes

Servings: 6

Ingredients:

- 4 tbsp. of nut butter

- 1 stick of unsalted butter

- 1 oz. of unsweetened dark chocolate

- 1/3 cup of stevia/monk fruit

- 2 tbsp. of heavy cream

Kitchen Equipment:

- muffin tin

- microwave

Directions:

1. Prepare a muffin tin with cupcake liner paper.

2. Melt the butter and chocolate in the microwave (checking at 30-second intervals).

3. Stir in the rest of the fixings.

4. Evenly distribute into the prepared tins and freeze for 30 minutes to an hour.

5. Gently tap the pan to remove.

Nutrition:

Net Carbohydrates: 1g - **Protein Counts:** 2g - **Total Fats:** 26g

44. BROWNIES

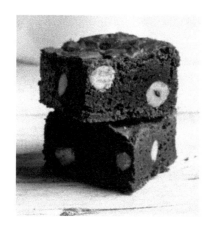

Preparation Time: 10 minutes

Cooking Time: 30 minutes

Servings: 12

Ingredients:

- ¼ tsp. of salt
- ¾ cup of cocoa powder
- 1 tsp. of vanilla extract
- ½ tsp. of baking soda
- 1 1/3 cups of almond flour
- 2/3 cup of coconut oil (separated)
- 2 eggs
- ½ cup of hot water
- 1 cup of stevia sugar substitute

Kitchen Equipment:

- oven
- 8-inch pan
- kitchen knife

Directions:

1. Heat your oven to 350 degrees F before you start.
2. Next, prepare an 8" pan by greasing it with coconut oil.
3. Get a medium bowl and throw your baking soda and cocoa powder into it.

Recipes from Keto

45.PEANUT BUTTER GRANOLA

Preparation Time: 10 minutes

Cooking Time: 40 minutes

Servings: 12

Ingredients:

- 2 cups of almonds
- 2 cups of pecans
- 1 cup of shredded coconut
- ¼ cup of sunflower seeds
- ¼ cup of water
- ¼ cup of butter
- 1/3 cup of sweetener
- 1/3 cup of vanilla protein powder
- 1/3 cup of peanut butter

Kitchen Equipment:

- oven
- parchment paper
- baking tray
- blender
- bowl

Directions:

1. Preheat your oven at 150 degrees Celsius.
2. Use parchment paper for lining a large baking tray.
3. Add pecans and almonds in a blender. Process for 2 minutes.
4. Combine processed mixture with sweetener, coconut, vanilla protein powder, and sunflower seeds.
5. Melt butter along with peanut butter in a bowl.
6. Add melted butter mixture over the mixture of nuts. Mix well.
7. Spread the nut mixture on the baking tray evenly.
8. Bake for 30 minutes.

Nutrition: Calories: 335.9 - **Protein:** 10.6g - **Fat:** 31.2g

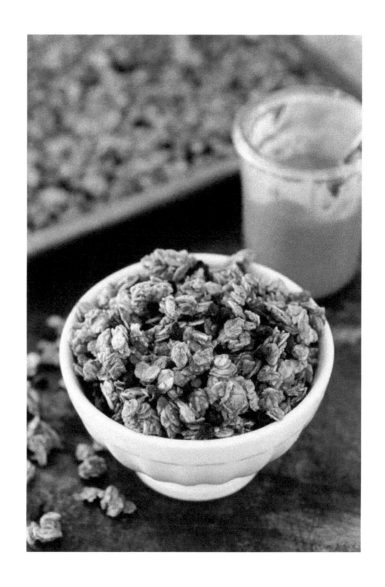

46. COCONUT PORRIDGE

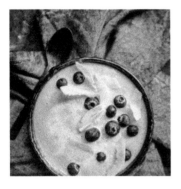

Preparation Time: 5 minutes

Cooking Time: 13 minutes

Servings: 6

Ingredients:

- 1 cup of shredded coconut (unsweetened)

- 2 cups of coconut milk (unsweetened and full-fat)

- 2 2/3 cups of water

- ¼ cup of coconut flour

- ¼ cup of psyllium husks

- 1 tsp. of vanilla extract, unsweetened

- ½ tsp. of cinnamon

- ¼ tsp. of nutmeg

- 30 drops of stevia (liquid)

- 20 drops of monk fruit sweetener (liquid)

Kitchen Equipment:

- instant pot

Directions:

1. Switch on the instant pot, select the 'sauté/simmer' button, once hot stir in the coconut and cook for 3 minutes or more until toasted.

2. Stir in water and milk, and press the 'keep warm' button.

3. Close the instant pot, then click the 'manual' button, press '+/-' to set cooking time to 10 minutes and click at high-pressure setting; when the pressure builds in the pot, the timer will start.

4. When the instant pot start ringing, click the 'keep warm' button, release pressure naturally

for 10 minutes, then gradually release the pressure and open the pot.

5. Add remaining ingredients, stir well and serve.

Nutrition:

Calories: 303 - **Fat:** 25g - **Protein:** 3g

47. BACON AND ZUCCHINI MUFFINS

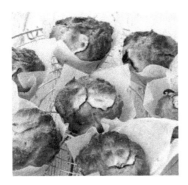

Preparation Time: 10 minutes

Cooking Time: 35 minutes

Servings: 8

Ingredients:

- 2 cups of grated zucchini

- 1 green onion (chopped)

- 2 thyme sprigs leaves removed

- ½ cup of coconut flour

- 7 eggs (pastured)

- ½ tsp. of salt

- 1 tsp. of ground turmeric

- 5 slices of bacon (pastured, diced)

- 1 tsp. of baking powder

- ½ tbsp. of apple cider vinegar

- 1 scoop of collagen peptides

Kitchen Equipment:

- oven

- medium frying pan

- silicon muffin tray

- wire rack

- freezer bag

- foil

Directions:

1. Prepare the oven at 350 degrees F and wait until muffins are ready to bake.

2. Take a medium frying pan, place it over medium heat, add bacon pieces, and cook for 3 to 5 minutes until crispy.

3. Then transfer cooked bacon in a large bowl, add remaining

ingredients and stir until well combined.

4. Take an eight cups silicon muffin tray, grease the cups with avocado oil and then evenly scoop the prepared batter in them.

5. Situate the muffin tray into the oven and bake the muffins for 30 minutes or until thoroughly cooked and the top is nicely golden brown.

6. When done, take out muffins from the tray and cool on the wire rack.

7. Place muffins in a large freezer bag or wrap each muffin with a foil and store them in the refrigerator for four days or in the freezer for up to 3 months.

8. When ready to serve, microwave muffins for 45 seconds to 1 minute or until thoroughly heated.

Nutrition:

Calories: 104 - **Fat:** 7.2g - **Protein:** 7.9g

48. PRETZELS

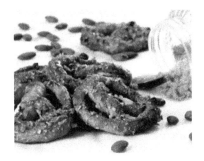

Preparation Time: 10 minutes

Cooking Time: 12 minutes

Servings: 6

Ingredients:

- 1 ½ cup of almond flour (blanched)

- ½ tsp. of coconut sugar

- 1 tbsp. of baking powder

- ¼ tsp. of xanthan gum

- 2 ¼ tsp. of dry yeast (active)

- ¼ cup of water (lukewarm)

- 2 eggs (pastured, beaten)

- 3 cups of mozzarella cheese (full-fat, shredded)

- 2 oz. of cream cheese (full-fat, cubed)

- 1 tsp. of salt

Kitchen Equipment:

- food processor

- heatproof bowl

- microwave

- baking sheet

- parchment paper

Directions:

1. Transfer the yeast in a small bowl, add sugar, pour in water, stir until just mixed allow it rest at a warm place for 10 minutes or until frothy.

2. Then pour the yeast mixture in a food

processor, add flour, xanthan gums, eggs, and baking powder and pulse for 1 to 2 minutes or until well combined.

3. Take a heatproof bowl, add cream cheese and m o z z a r e l l a   a n d microwave for 2 minutes or until melted, stirring every 30 seconds until smooth.

4. Add melted cheese into the processed flour mixture and continue blending until the dough comes together, continue scrape the mixture from the sides of the blender.

5. Transfer the dough into a bowl and then place it in the refrigerator for 20 minutes or until chilled.

6. Meanwhile, preheat the oven at 400 degrees F and let preheat.

7. Take out the chilled dough from the refrigerator, then divide the dough into six sections and shape each section into a bowl, using oiled hands.

8. Simultaneously, first, roll the section into an 18-inches long log, then take one end, loop it around and down across the bottom and loop the other end, in the same manner, crossing over the first loop to form a pretzel.

9. Prepare remaining pretzels in the same manner and place them on a baking sheet lined with parchment sheet.

10. Sprinkle salt over pretzels, pressing down lightly, then place the baking sheet into the oven and bake pretzels

for 10 to 12 minutes until nicely golden.

11. When done, cool the pretzels at room temperature, then keep them in a large plastic bag and freeze it for 3 months or store them in the refrigerator for up to a week.

12. When ready to serve, bake the pretzels at 400 degrees F for 6 to 7 minutes until hot.

Nutrition:

Calories: 370 - **Fat:** 28g - **Protein:** 23g

49. KETO COCONUT FLOUR EGG MUFFIN

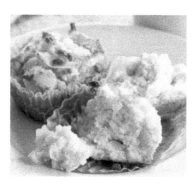

Preparation Time: 5 minutes

Cooking Time: 10 minutes

Servings: 2

Ingredients:

- 1 organic egg (large-sized)

- 2 teaspoons coconut flour or as required

- A pinch of baking soda

- 1 tablespoon of coconut oil (to coat)

- Salt (to taste)

Kitchen Equipment:

- oven

- large-sized coffee mug

Directions:

1. Preheat your oven to 400°F.

2. Lightly coat a large-sized coffee mug or ramekin dish with some coconut oil.

3. Using a fork, mix the entire ingredients together and make sure no lumps remain.

4. Bake for 10 to 12 minutes, until cooked through.

5. Cut in half, serve immediately and enjoy.

Nutrition:

Calories: 48 - **Total Fat:** 3.9g - **Total Carbohydrates:** 1.7g

50. BROCCOLI CHEDDAR CHEESE MUFFINS

Preparation Time: 10 minutes

Cooking Time: 15 minutes

Servings: 6

Ingredients:

- 2/3 cup of cheddar cheese

- ¼ teaspoon of garlic powder

- ¾ cup of broccoli, steamed and chopped (fresh or frozen and thawed)

- ¼ teaspoon of dried thyme

Kitchen Equipment:

- oven

- large-sized mixing bowl

- muffin tins

Directions:

1. Preheat your oven to 400°F.

2. Combine the thyme with garlic powder in a large-sized mixing bowl until combined well and then, stir in the cheddar and broccoli.

3. Evenly split the mixture into the muffin tins (with 6 cups) filling each cup approximately 2/3 full.

4. Sprinkle with more of cheddar on top, if desired and then, bake until completely set, for 12 to 15 minutes.

5. Serve immediately and enjoy.

Nutrition:

Calories: 33 - **Total Fat:** 4.2g - **Total Carbohydrates:** 1.8g

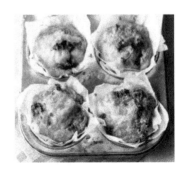

KETOGENIC DIET FOOD LIST

FATS & OILS

- Fatty Fish
- Animal Fat
- Tallow
- Avocados
- Egg Yolks
- Macadamia Nuts
- Butter/Ghee
- Real Mayonnaise
- Coconut Butter
- Cocoa Butter
- Olive Oil
- Coconut Oil
- Avocado Oil
- Macadamia Oil

PROTEIN

Bacon & Sausage
Beef
Fish and shellfish
Nut butter*
Organ meat
Pork
Poultry
Whole eggs

DAIRY

Butter
Cheese
Ghee
Yogurt
Heavy cream
Sour cream

VEGETABLES

- Asparagus
- Bok choy
- Broccoli
- Cauliflower
- Celery
- Cucumber
- Endive
- Kale
- Leafy greens
- Lettuce
- Mushrooms
- Radishes
- Spinach
- Sprouts (alfalfa, bean)
- Swiss chard
- Yellow Squash & zucchini
- Turnip
- Cabbage
- Onions
- Beetroot
- Kolrabi
- Bell Pepper

DRINKS

Water
Bone broth
Coffee (black or bulletproof
Nut milks
Tea

FRUIT

Avocado
Blackberries
Blueberries
Lemon Juice
Raspberries
Strawberries

MY RECIPES HOMEMADE

Recipe:_____

Rating: ☆☆☆☆☆ Difficulty: ☆☆☆☆☆ Prep Time:_____ Cook Time:

Ingredients:_____

_____

_____

_____

Cooking Instructions:_____

_____

_____

_____

_____

_____

_____

_____

Thoughts and Notes:

_____

_____

Recipe:_____

Rating: ☆☆☆☆☆ Difficulty: ☆☆☆☆☆ Prep Time:_____ Cook Time:_____

Ingredients:_____

_____

_____

_____

_____

Cooking Instructions:_____

_____

_____

_____

_____

_____

_____

_____

Thoughts and Notes:

_____

_____

_____

Recipe: _____

Rating: ☆☆☆☆☆ Difficulty: ☆☆☆☆☆ Prep Time: _____ Cook Time: _____

Ingredients: _____

_____

_____

_____

Cooking Instructions: _____

_____

_____

_____

_____

_____

_____

Thoughts and Notes: _____

_____

_____

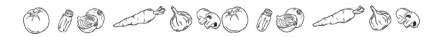

Recipe:_____

Rating: ☆☆☆☆☆ Difficulty: ☆☆☆☆☆ Prep Time: _____ Cook Time: _____

Ingredients:_____

_____

_____

_____

Cooking Instructions:_____

_____

_____

_____

_____

_____

_____

_____

Thoughts and Notes:

_____

_____

Recipe: _____

Rating: ☆☆☆☆☆ *Difficulty:* ☆☆☆☆☆ *Prep Time:* _____ *Cook Time:* _____

Ingredients: _____

_____

_____

_____

Cooking Instructions: _____

_____

_____

_____

_____

_____

_____

Thoughts and Notes:

_____

_____

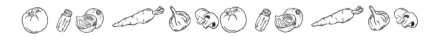

Recipe: _____

Rating: ☆☆☆☆☆ Difficulty: ☆☆☆☆☆ Prep Time: _____   Cook Time: _____

Ingredients: _____

_____

_____

_____

Cooking Instructions: _____

_____

_____

_____

_____

_____

_____

Thoughts and Notes: _____

_____

_____

Recipe:

Rating: ☆☆☆☆☆ Difficulty: ☆☆☆☆☆ Prep Time: Cook Time:

Ingredients:

Cooking Instructions:

Thoughts and Notes:

Recipe: _____

Rating: ☆☆☆☆☆ Difficulty: ☆☆☆☆☆ Prep Time: _____ Cook Time: _____

Ingredients: _____

_____

_____

_____

_____

Cooking Instructions: _____

_____

_____

_____

_____

_____

_____

_____

Thoughts and Notes: _____

_____

_____

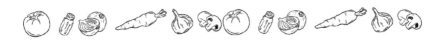

*Recipe:*_____

Rating: ☆☆☆☆☆ *Difficulty:* ☆☆☆☆☆ *Prep Time:*   *Cook Time:*

*Ingredients:*_____

_____

_____

_____

*Cooking Instructions:*_____

_____

_____

_____

_____

_____

_____

Thoughts and Notes:

_____

_____

Recipe:

Rating: ☆☆☆☆☆ Difficulty: ☆☆☆☆☆ Prep Time: Cook Time:

Ingredients:

Cooking Instructions:

Thoughts and Notes:

Recipe: _____

Rating: ☆☆☆☆☆ Difficulty: ☆☆☆☆☆ Prep Time: _____ Cook Time: _____

Ingredients: _____

_____

_____

_____

Cooking Instructions: _____

_____

_____

_____

_____

_____

_____

Thoughts and Notes: _____

_____

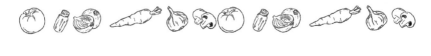

Recipe: _____

Rating: ☆☆☆☆☆ Difficulty: ☆☆☆☆☆ Prep Time: _____   Cook Time: _____

Ingredients: _____

_____

_____

_____

Cooking Instructions: _____

_____

_____

_____

_____

_____

_____

Thoughts and Notes: _____

_____

_____

Recipe: _____

Rating: ☆☆☆☆☆ Difficulty: ☆☆☆☆☆ Prep Time: _____ Cook Time: _____

Ingredients: _____

_____

_____

_____

_____

Cooking Instructions: _____

_____

_____

_____

_____

_____

_____

Thoughts and Notes: _____

_____

_____

CPSIA information can be obtained
at www.ICGtesting.com
Printed in the USA
BVHW091729110521
607043BV00010B/1863